Primal Walk

Margo,
Keep on your toes!!
yes pal,
GS

Greg Shim

ISBN: 1543295916
ISBN 13: 9781543295917
Library of Congress Control Number: 2017902885
LCCN Imprint Name: Castle Rock, CO

This book is dedicated to the thousands of people who have helped me refine the ideas I put forth here.

Also to my daughter, who has given me inspiration to find a way to keep her healthy and strong.

And, most of all, to my wife, who has been by my side for more than twenty years as I've tried (and continue to try) to piece together what life is all about!

CHAPTER 1

Don't Be a Swayback!

Primal walking is not easy. It's a discipline that takes more than double the calories than what we've come to consider "normal" walking and more than a bit of mindfulness. But as with any discipline, it brings about a better connection between your mind and body and, in doing so, makes a better connection between you and the world around you.

We're mammals, and like most mammals, we get around by walking. When we see mammals walking and sprinting about in the wild, we see grace and strength. We rarely, if ever, see slumped and swaybacked mammals, as they tend to die off quickly or be killed and eaten—which brings me to the point of this book. Lacking large predators to kill us and eat us, modernized humans have become slaves to convenience; in the United States, we have become a swayback nation.

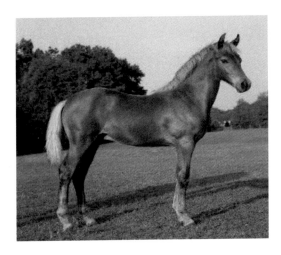 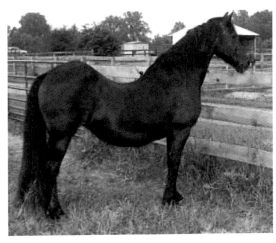

Look at the two horses above and ask yourself, "Which horse am I?" For most people in developed countries, the answer to the question is the second horse, but the first horse is what we can be.

That may sound a bit extreme, but let's talk about what a swayback is. Any mammal can be a swayback. Swaybacks lack stability, and their frames fail. The horse on the right is a swayback. It's standing on its bones. Notice how it has its hoof directly under its shoulder in a straight line. There's very little muscle tone, and, since the horse lacks stability, its back and joints are failing. The horse on the left has great tone and stability. Notice how the shoulder is still over the hoof, but there's a backward bend at the fetlock (what would be your ankle). This book is about bringing out the stability of the first horse in your own body.

A swayback mammal relies on its bones to hold it up while the stable mammal (no pun intended) relies on its connective tissue and deep core to keep it upright and moving. The cover of this book shows sticks being held together by tension in connecting wires. The proper word for this would be tensegrity ("tensional integrity"), coined by the architect Buckminster Fuller back in the sixties, but I think it would be more commonly thought of as stability. Those wires are your connective tissue, and the sticks are your bones. The stronger the wires, the more the "bones" float, and the more stable the structure—your body!

If you're standing on your heels and heel-striking when you walk, you're a swayback. As a swayback, you have a much greater chance of becoming swaybacked, having a weak core, and having your joints fail.

Since this book is about bringing out stability, let's see where you stand (or sit) with regard to deep core stability. One way you can test your core strength is by sitting in a chair and having another person either hold your forehead with two fingers (or your chest, if your neck has pain). If you can't push forward slowly and stand up, your core isn't as strong as you think it is.

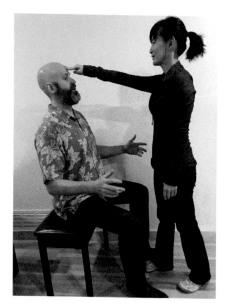 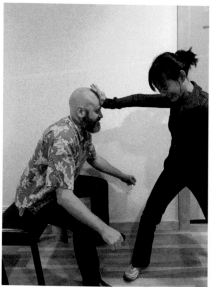

If your core is truly strong, standing up against this pressure shouldn't be much work.

Most people whom I test in the United States don't pass the two-finger test; many can't even move through a pinky on the forehead! Seven years ago, you could have held me down with a pinky, but now I can push through someone leaning on my forehead. All that core strength was achieved just by changing the way I walked, and I went from being a five-foot-ten heel-striker (203 pounds at my heaviest) to a five-foot-eleven forefoot-walker!

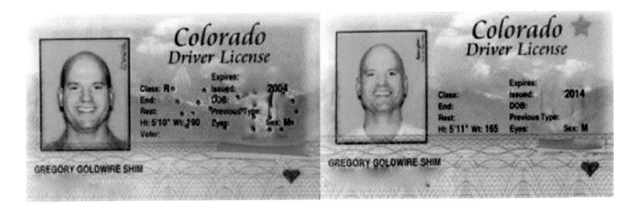

If you're like me, you need concrete evidence, so let's do a couple of tests, and you can prove to yourself that the way you walk may be a hindrance. First, check yourself on how you walk and how you stand. If you wear your heels down on your shoe, you're a heel-striker, and you're in for a treat! If the front of your shoe is worn and the heel looks new, you're most likely a solid forefoot-striker, and this book might not be as dramatic for you personally. However, I've met several forefoot-strikers who still are swaybacks. So even if you're a forefoot-striker, the rest of your body might not have the proper form for full-body stability, so don't quit reading quite yet.

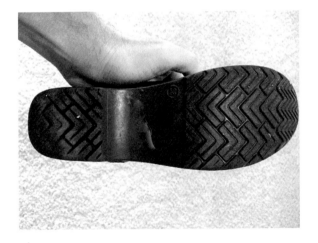
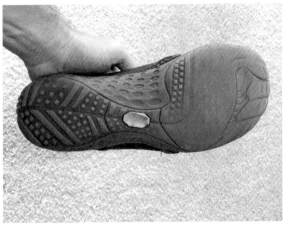

If you're like most people in the United States, your shoes are worn down on the heels, so you lack your full stability. A person who is a swayback is missing that potential, as strength comes from stability. As Socrates said, "No person has the right to be an amateur in the matter of physical training. It is a shame for someone to grow old without seeing the beauty and strength of which the body is capable."

3

CHAPTER 2

How Not to Be a Swayback!

To find your nonswayback potential, stand on your heels (most likely how you usually stand) and put one arm out. Next, have someone place his or her hand on your wrist (not your hand) and slowly press down. The person shouldn't have too much trouble forcing your arm down, and you get the "pleasure" of feeling your shoulder muscles as they strain to do a job they weren't meant to do.

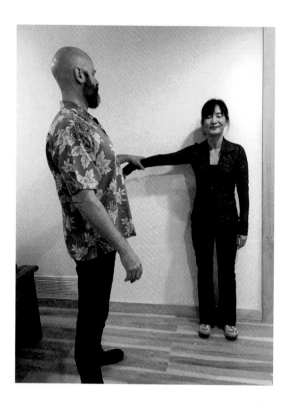
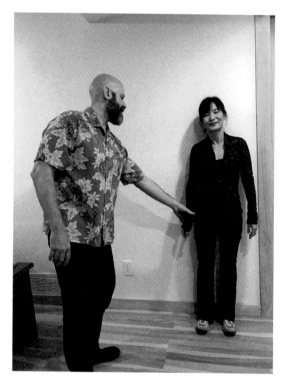

Now let's repeat that exercise, but with your full stability in play. First, put 99 percent of your weight on the balls of your feet, or just go up on the balls of your feet a bit—you're going to feel like you're leaning slightly forward. Your hips should be over the balls of your feet and your knees should not be locked. Next, lift your breastbone up; in other words, stick out your chest while simultaneously bringing your head back (don't worry about the shoulders), and make sure your chin is pulled in. You should feel your entire abdomen get flatter and tighter—don't deliberately tighten your core; just feel how everything naturally gets tight. The higher you go on your toes, the more stability you create. More stability equals greater strength (but you don't have to walk around high on your tiptoes).

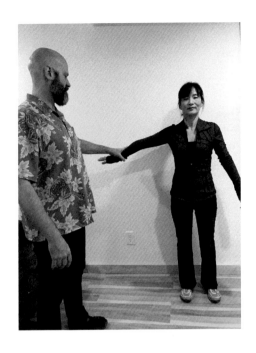 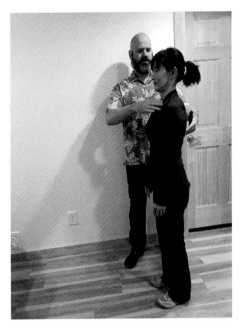

If you're on the balls of your feet, with your chest up and your head pulled back with the chin in, you should feel considerably more strength as you put your full stability to use. With time and primal walking, your stability and strength will increase dramatically. The muscles help, but it's the combined stability of connective tissue, muscles, and bones that gives us our strength. If you're still not feeling the improved stability throughout the arm, pay attention to your shoulders—they should not be pulled back. The shoulders should be in line with your ears and relaxed. When pressure is applied to your wrist, see if you can feel the pull all the way into your opposite leg. Most people, having lived much of their lives as swaybacks, tend to think that pulling the shoulders back helps with posture. In reality, it just helps with making your upper back and neck tight.

As an acupuncturist who practices Traditional Chinese Medicine (TCM), I don't spend as much time treating a single body part as I do treating the whole body. After six years and fifteen thousand patient visits or so, an even larger picture of what the body is began to emerge, and the Chinese saying, "The best practitioners have the fewest patients," began to finally sink in. This book is a result of a desire to live up to that saying.

In TCM we have a concept called Zheng Qi. My teachers could never tell me what it was; all they would do was translate it literally into English. They'd say that Zheng Qi means "correct vitality," "upright vitality," or "chest vitality." They'd also say that all the rest of our vitality stems from this core vitality. If I pressed for more information, they'd change the subject, and that would be the end of the conversation. Looking back, I realize that they were swaybacks like everyone else in the classroom, including myself. It's very difficult to say what something is if you have little or no experience with it.

We talk about yin and yang in TCM as well. You can think of the connective tissues and muscles as being soft, pliable "yin" and the hard, strong bone as "yang."

When these are used together, we are stronger than when we use either alone. If you're only standing on your bones, you're not using the whole system, and you're moving faster toward yin-and-yang separation. As the TCM saying goes, when yin and yang separate, there is death.

On the bottom of your foot is an acupuncture point called Kidney 1, or, Bubbling Spring. This is a point for dumping bad energy and pulling in good energy. When you stand correctly on the balls of your feet, you are standing on Bubbling Spring. Traditional Chinese Medicine states that if you study the ancient texts, all the information you need for practicing good medicine is already there—and in this case, I agree! Good posture starts in the feet!

When you stand with stability, you can feel the uprightness of your body. You can feel the strength of your core and see how correct your body looks. And with your breastbone lifted, you are giving vitality to your chest and breath. By practicing primal walking, we can cultivate Zheng Qi and cultivate our true beauty and strength potential.

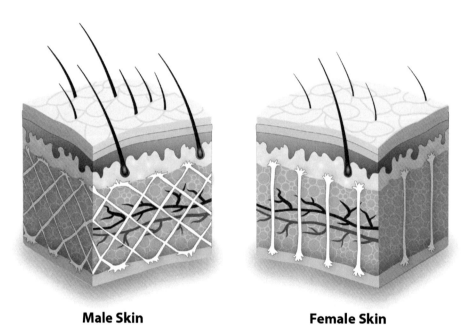

Male Skin　　　　　　　　**Female Skin**

As you can see in the image above, men are naturally more durable than women. Think of all the times a woman has struggled with a jar lid, and then a man just pops it off. Women are literally tearing their skin while men have a built in mesh. This is why it's so important for girls and women to cultivate Zheng Qi - think of Zheng Qi as posture. The better your posture, the better you strengthen your connective tissue!

CHAPTER 3

Details

Now that we have the foundation, let's move into a primal walk. Most people in the modern world are heel-strikers—it's just more convenient to walk that way. According to one study (Cunningham et al. 2010), it takes 53 percent less energy to heel-strike. So why would I want to change my walk? For starters, if I'm using 53 percent less energy just walking around, that's 53 percent fewer calories burned in my day!

More importantly, primal walking gives you an amazing core! With a strong core, women better retain continence, and men can better avoid erectile dysfunction. Just google "lack of core strength and incontinence" or "lack of core strength and erectile dysfunction," and you'll be bombarded by a multitude of research. Primal walking will pump blood to your pelvic area, where the blood can nourish all the organs and muscles.

If you've ever been around children learning to walk, you'll notice they stay on their toes. When I was growing up, I kept this forefoot walk for many years, slowly changing my walk in response to how the adults were walking around me. By elementary school, I was a full-fledged heel-striker, and I joined my peers in teasing and name-calling the kids who kept their natural walk. One boy in particular was teased mercilessly, but by the time he was in middle school, nobody teased him anymore; he was stronger and more powerful than all the heel-strikers around him.

For those who would jump up and start spouting that toe-walking is pathologic, I would agree wholeheartedly that there are disorders for which toe-walking is a problem. But we won't be toe-walking; we'll be forefoot-striking on the balls of our feet. So let's get into the forefoot walk, and then you can judge for yourself which path you want to take.

First, let's see where we want to hit. Pick up your leg and let your foot hang out in front of you. Now, pull your toes up toward your knee. Next, point your toes down toward the ground. Repeat this toes-up and toes-down movement twice more, and then pull your toes up and hold for three seconds.

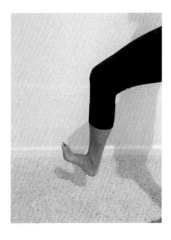 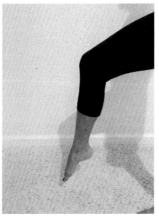 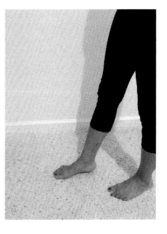

Now relax the foot and gently place it down in front of you. That's where you want to set your foot. Your steps will be shorter than when you heel-strike, but with time you'll be walking just as fast (or faster) as you were with the heel walk. Later on, I'll show how to maximize your deep core to walk with even more stability and speed, but for now, just keep the steps short and practice until it feels at least a little natural (at forty-three, it took eight months to feel fully natural for me).

Now that we have foot placement and a shorter step, it's time to address that swayback sported by many people in the modern world as they age—and by more and more teens I've seen recently. Note that because we have two legs instead of four like most other mammals, our sway will be in more than one place along our back.

Once you have nailed the stepping down, the next thing to do is to draw the head back until the ear is in line with the shoulder while lifting your chest. Just focus on the head right now, because the shoulders aren't involved with posture. I usually touch the middle of the back with one hand and the sternum with the other to help my patients feel the lift. Now lift the sternum up, keeping the head drawn back. You're now on your way to your true height! It took two years, but I eventually gained an inch! Gravity is always trying to pull you into the earth, and it will win one day—but don't let it be today! Even though you won't gain the two inches that astronaut Scott Kelly gained without gravity, you can still gain some by fighting gravity with your walk.

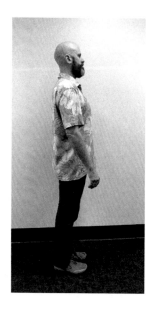 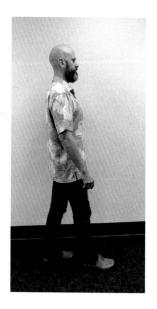

Notice your head alignment as you forefoot-strike. As you can see, the alignment of the ear never changes when you forefoot-strike! Practice with a book on your head. Back in the day, people did this on a regular basis, but now it's just a memory of etiquette school.

One way that I help people find their proper alignment is with a wall. Keeping on the ball of your foot, put your heels, your bottom, your back, and the back of your head against the wall. Once you're in position and keeping your alignment, shift your upper body – head, shoulders, back, and hips move as one unit - so your hips are over the balls of your feet. If you're too swayback to get your head against the wall, keep trying everyday! Deswaybacking does not happen fast, and to rid yourself of all your swayback tissue, you're looking at 5 to 10 years – but it's worth it!!!

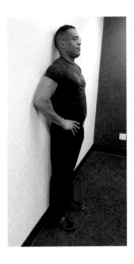 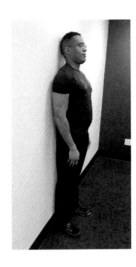 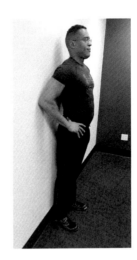

So let's see what happens when you heel-strike. Look at that forward head position (and the paunch)—and age them by sixty years! If your head weighs sixteen pounds, it pulls at thirty-two pounds with your head forward and pulls at an astounding sixty-four pounds when you are a full-blown swayback! I'd be grouchy, too, with that much weight pulling on my spine.

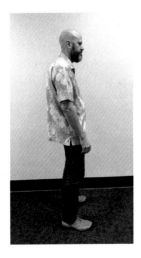 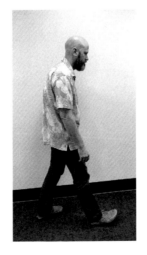 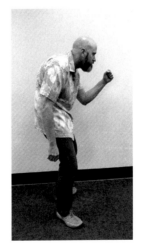

Get off my lawn!

CHAPTER 4

Added Bonuses

Calves

Now that you've started your primal walk, you'll notice other benefits. First, you get powerful calves. They may take a year or so to develop, but if you're forefoot-striking, they will. Here's why—try it on yourself! First, press into your inner calf.

Notice how the calf doesn't fire when you land on your heel. Now forefoot-strike—that's using your body correctly!

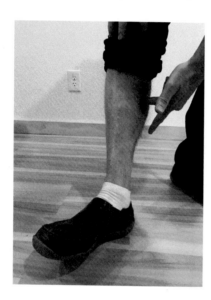 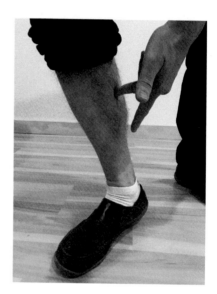

When you forefoot-strike, you're using your leg the way it was meant to be used. Those calves aren't just for good looks, though; they're also pumping blood and lymph (cell sewage) back to the heart with every step. It's almost like having two extra hearts whenever you're walking! Conversely, when you're standing and striking on your heel, you can feel the muscles contract in the front of the shin. Those muscles (especially extensor digitorum longus) contribute to hammer toes. When you're on the ball of your foot, those front muscles are relaxed.

Iliotibial Band

Research has come out over the last several years that points to obesity as more of an inflammatory condition rather than just an outcome of people sitting and shoving fast food down their gullets (although there is that). If I overuse a tendon, it becomes inflamed. If I end up with chronic inflammation in an area, it may swell up a bit.

With that in mind, let's take a look at the Iliotibial (IT) Band, the big, wide white band of connective tissue that ties in the knee to the hips and back. If I overuse or misuse it, it's going to get angry and can become inflamed. But don't take my word for it; see for yourself! Grab your leg with your hand over your IT band. Step down on your heel and feel that cable/IT band pop right out! Now land on your forefoot and feel how the whole leg engages.

Overuse of the IT band from heel-striking carries a very distinctive look once the area becomes inflamed. Notice in the picture below how there's swelling over the IT band (saddlebags), calves are underdeveloped, and because of lack of stability, the ankles are falling in on themselves.

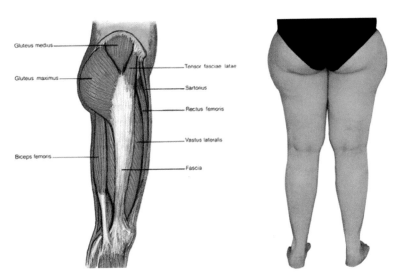

Unlike the swayback horse shown at the beginning of the book, you have the ability to change your walk and re-create the stability you strove so hard to achieve as a child learning to walk. If even a child is desperately working on stability and core strength, when is it a good time to stop working on stability and strength?
Don't be a swayback!

Core and Abdomen

Standing in a way that enhances your stability—99 percent of your weight on your forefeet (a.k.a. the balls of your feet), head drawn back, chin in, and sternum raised—feel your stomach. Even though you're relaxed, your abdomen is tight. Make sure you don't lock your knees!

Now press your fingers into your abdomen, and while you're holding your fingers there, start walking in place. Do you feel that? That's your deep core being engaged and contracting, effectively working out your core whenever you're standing or primal walking. You can periodically check yourself by pressing into your stomach as you walk—if you can feel the contractions as you walk, you're doing it right. This all happens without effort, so don't walk around consciously contracting and uncontracting your abs.

Over time, all that connective tissue being engaged will get stronger and stronger. The more you forefoot-strike and forefoot-stand, the stronger and more resilient you become.

You'll feel some discomfort as you develop this walk, so make sure you take some time to keep yourself feeling good. Massage therapists, personal trainers, chiropractors, physical therapists, and acupuncturists are your friends!

Say Good-bye to the Monkey Mind

Stand on the ball of your foot with good posture. What are you thinking about? Probably the same thing I think of after seven years of forefoot-standing: standing! Now walk with a forefoot-strike. What are you thinking about? Walking! This walk has been called the "Walk of the Immortals" in some TCM circles, and for good reasons. You stay tall, and your head isn't filled with drama. A clear and calm mind is priceless.

Greater Bioresiliency

Our bodies develop greater bioresiliency with this gait as well. Our core connective tissue strengthens from use, just like the rest of our body does from proper exercise. We can also avoid injury—much like the runners did in Daniel Lieberman's Harvard study (Lieberman et al. 2010). The heel-strikers had 100 percent more injuries than the forefoot-strikers! That's a pretty big difference. Think of hitting the sculpture on the front cover of this book with a rubber hammer; the vibration would just spread out through the wires and "bones." On your heels, you get hit, and the damage is right where you've been struck. As we move away from stability, we're more prone to damage. I've often wondered what sets the stage for so many more concussions these days, and the lack of stability and resilience in modern kids' bodies is one possible answer (lack of piezoelectric current could be another – but we'll get to that later).

CHAPTER 5

Applications

So how can you put your new knowledge to work? Even though you may just be starting to walk this way, it's not too early to put stability to work.

Core123

First and foremost is what I lovingly refer to as the Core123 with my patients. This is one of my favorite things to teach because it can be very beneficial and can help people with low back pain without me even touching them. The first thing to do is a Kegel exercise. If you don't know what that is, just tighten the muscles you would tighten when you have to pee badly and hold the tension.

Second, tighten your bottom sphincter (not the butt cheeks)—pretend you have some bad gas, but you're in front of polite company. When you hold the Kegel and the sphincter lock, you should feel your whole pelvic floor rise up a little inside you.

Lastly, bear down like you're constipated and push your stomach out—not all the way out, but definitely some. This really activates the transverse abdominals, which protects your lower back. I know people love to suck their stomachs in, but unless you've done lots of advanced training, it's very difficult to keep your transverse abs engaged while you suck your stomach in.

Don't believe me? Try this: Press on your abs and your lower back muscles, standing with stability—that is, weight on the balls of your feet, chest and breastbone raised up, head back over the shoulders, and chin pulled in.

Next, do the Core123 - or Kegel, sphincter lock, and bear down. Feel those back muscles push out? Your back is now protected. Now suck in your stomach. If you did the Core123 correctly, your back, upon sucking in your stomach, would become mushy, and you'd just be asking for back pain.

The Core123 can be used to increase stability while you're walking as well. If you want a longer stride, just do the Core123. The harder you do it, the faster you can go! Here's a fun fact: doing the Core123 in a stability stance while way up on your forefoot (tiptoe) maximizes stability! If you're sitting and need to lift something, make sure you do the Core123 to protect your back and give the rest of your body the stability it needs to move the weight you're lifting.

Pinkies under the Heels

I like this technique when helping others get a feel for how they should stand in activities, although it can be a bit painful on my pinkies (notice my wife's smile).

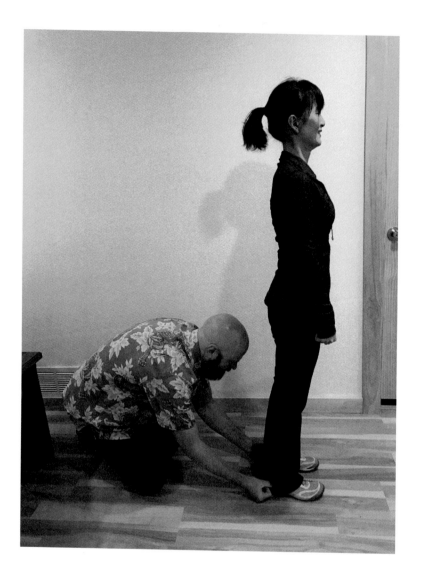

First, stand with stability. Next, have someone put their pinkies under your heels. Last, don't hurt them! Squatting, singing, shooting, stretching, golfing, and standing are all actions that can and should be done in this position. Pretty much at any given time I'm on my feet, someone could comfortably put their pinkies under my heels and feel no discomfort on their fingers.

CHAPTER 6

Getting There Faster

My patients spend sixty to one hundred twenty minutes at my clinic when they come to see me. I hop back and forth between two rooms and generally see one or two people an hour. I've had about thirty-seven thousand patient visits over the last fifteen years, so I've learned a few "trickniques" that might be of use to you.

Doorjamb Stretch

There are lots of connective tissue knots that build up in the body from misuse. The IT bands and hip rotators take a beating when we heel-strike. As you change your walk, you can use this stretch before bed to help open the hips.

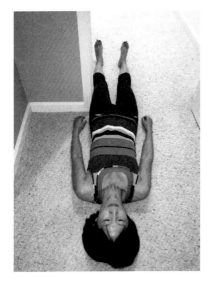 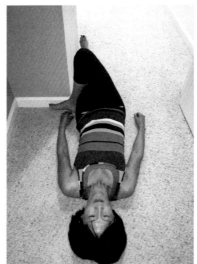 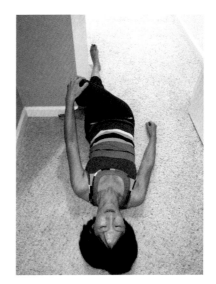

- First, lie on the floor and press your thigh or knee into a doorjamb or something heavy.

- Next, bring your opposite foot over and lock it into the wall with the whole foot (yes, even the heel—you're not standing). Now use the opposite hand to pull the knee across your body.

Hold this for about two minutes on each side before bed to keep those hips loose!

Modified Thoracic Bridges

This is a great way to improve your toe touches and to help gain the chest lift that's important to the forefoot gait. While you can google "thoracic bridges," I've developed a modified version to help you get to the full version. It can be done just about anywhere at any time.

Stand while holding on to something stable. This is our starting point. Release one hand and turn 180 degrees. Then turn and go back the same way you came to the starting point; now release the other hand, go the other way, and proceed the same way on the other side.

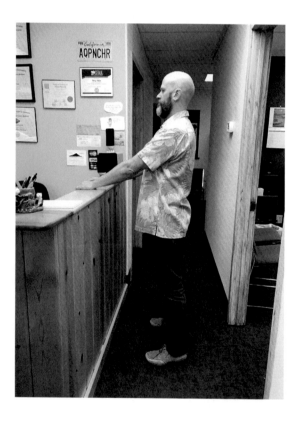 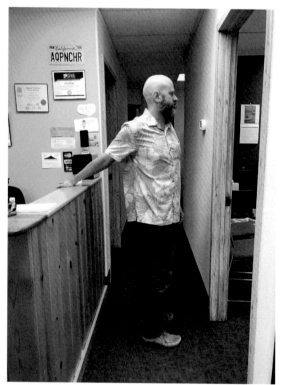

- Stand while holding on to something stable. This is our starting point.

- Release one hand and turn 180 degrees.

- Then turn and go back the same way you came to the starting point; now release the other hand, go the other way, and proceed the same way on the other side.

  Well done! You're ready for the tough part.

- Repeat the first step, but once you've turned 180 degrees, take the free arm and pull it across your chest as hard as you can while keeping the arm straight and stiff.

- Now press your hips forward, but not for too long. It's a mobility drill, not a stretch!

- Come back around and repeat with the other arm.

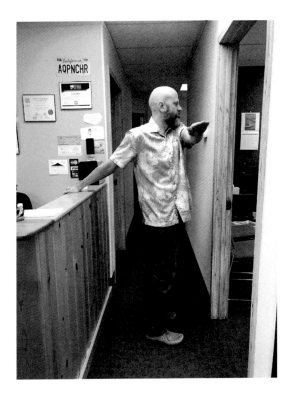 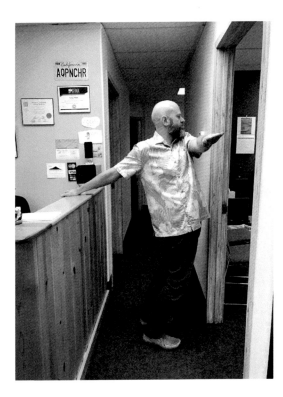

I like to do this mobility drill three times, especially when I first get out of bed, but you can do it as many times during the day as it feels good.

But remember—if it hurts, don't do it!

CHAPTER 7
Other Fun Things to Do

Walter Goodall George was an amazing British runner who set a mile-running record in 1886 that wasn't broken until the twentieth century. He had a technique in which he would work his way up to one hundred steps: the 100-Up! One can quickly learn the 100-Up, but it takes a while to master it.

Basically, in front of a large mirror, you primal-walk in place between two lines that are eighteen inches apart. Move with stability, raising your knees to hip level or as you're able, and moving your opposite hand, much as if you were marching. It is a slow, steady, methodical movement, and if you miss a step, falter, or step out of the lines, you're done for the day. Keep doing your perfect practice, and immediately stop for the day whenever it's not perfect.

Once you are able to do one hundred steps in place, you can move to the more advanced 100-Up. Instead of taking slow steps, you can increase the speed while still keeping the knees high and the form perfect. At this point, you're running in place, but if you falter, miss a step, or step out of the lines, you're done for the day. Keep it perfect and build up slowly, just as you should do your forefoot walk; you will avoid injury more readily by taking your time. Continuing to practice this walk and style of exercise will mean you're in it for the long haul!

CHAPTER 8

How We Got Here and Why Posture has Purpose!

I had a theory that our heel-striking walk developed in the United States because of our wealth. As you can see in this old cartoon, the poor must keep stability because their lives depend on it, and the rich can flaunt their heel-strike because they don't have to keep their strength and resiliency. But when was the last time you were chased by a pack of wolves? When was the last time you had to walk ten to fifteen miles on a daily basis for water and food? When was the last time you had to struggle in a field year after year because your ability to eat depended on getting a harvest?

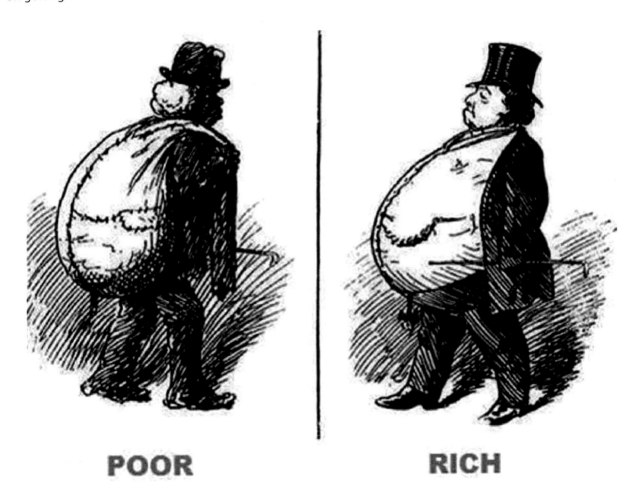

POOR   **RICH**

I've abandoned the wealth idea (even though there may be some truth to it) for one of pure convenience. It's simply too easy nowadays—53 percent easier!—to land on your heel. And if you're still not convinced, look at some old movies, such as A Trip to the Moon (1902) and see how people walk and run. They're all forefoot-striking! Remember when the hoboes in the Laurel and Hardy movies would put their feet on the table? The holes in their shoes were in the front! My older patients tell me that when they were young, they would wear holes in their shoes. Interestingly enough, they'd fold up newspaper pages and shove them to the front of their shoes, because that's where the holes were.

With the advent of the car, we acquired the ability to get food just by driving to a store. By the mid 1960s, most of the hardwood floors in offices had to be ripped out, because the kids born in the 1940s started working, and as heel strikers, they were denting the floors. Carpet was used instead, as it was much more comfortable to heel strike on a thick carpet. Airplanes also had to reengineer their floors to absorb the impact energy of people hitting their heels instead of the balls of their feet. And then in 1970, cushy heels for our shoes were invented, and we just became used to being able to heel-strike. By the early 1980s, cushioned heels became the norm and we've gotten weaker and sicker since then.

Still, the reasons for our heel-striking are not as important as getting back to walking in a way that promotes stability and strength. Interestingly enough, we've been heel-striking for so long now that we've come to admire the jutting chins and curvy bodies of swaybacked individuals. Culture isn't always correct when it comes to beauty combined with health!

So, what are the benefits of having purposeful posture? One of the most surprising benefits is that we generate more electricity when we have good posture than when we're swaybacks. When I first learned about this, it sounded like crazy talk to me, but let me give a few more details.

Have you ever used a grill lighter where you have to squeeze the trigger to get it to light? You have to squeeze fairly hard, and then it clicks, and voila – flame! The surprising part of this lighter is that you're squeezing on a piece of quartz with the trigger, and that strong squeeze, follow by a quick release, makes the quartz generate a very small electrical current called piezoelectric current. That little current arcs to metal on the grill lighter, and that electric arc ignites the lighter fluid. They use piezoelectric ceramic disks in shoes, as well, to make them light up – although they should be in the front of the shoe, and not the heel!

The crazy part is that collagen – connective tissue – is also piezoelectric. Piezo comes from Greek, "to squeeze", and unless you've got that tensional integrity (standing tall and on the ball of your foot), you're not engaging that squeeze. What's even more surprising is all those bazillions of little currents you generate from the piezoelectric effect of connective tissue drives growth of healthy tissue and helps regenerate the body. The better your posture and walk, the better your piezoelectric currents!

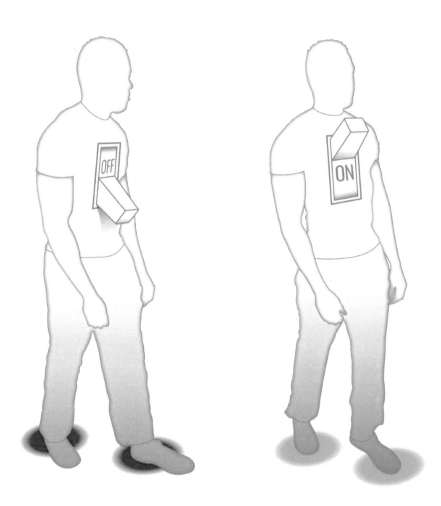

If you walk on your heels, you're creating biostatic shock (the forces that injure you in the Harvard running studies), and you're not making the currents that help keep you strong and healthy. When you do walk the way our ancestors did, you're strengthening your connective tissue and the benefits of that are enormous. Try thinking of body as a big bundle of connective tissue through which all this current is generated and flows. The better your connective tissue, the better it can house all the different tissues. The better the tissues are housed, the healthier you are.

Let's put some of these ideas together. The brain is 90% connective tissue, and if we look at when most modern people started heel striking in the West, we can see an ugly trend.

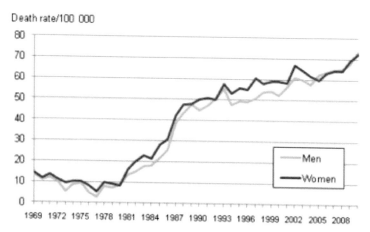

Figure 8. Age-standardised dementia mortality (incl. Alzheimer's disease) in 1969 to 2010 per 100,000 persons of the mean population

Death rate/100 000

Likewise, if you've ever taken a chicken bone and put it in vinegar, after about a week, it still looks like a bone, but now you can bend it easily. The vinegar, being a weak acid, has dissolved all the calcium out of the, "bone" and what's left is collagen – connective tissue! If we keep thinking of the body as a big bundle of connective tissue rather than parts, then this next chart (whose authors can't explain why the huge increase in osteoporosis related ankle fractures) is no surprise.

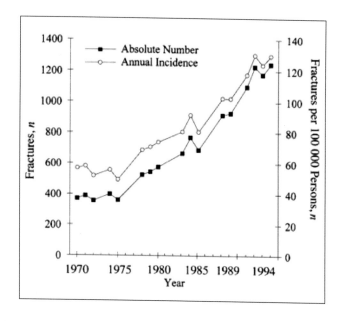

This graph shows rates of ankle fractures from osteoporosis. Weak piezoelectric currents from swaybacks don't allow the collagen to house the calcium, and so the bones become brittle. A different way to look at how the connective tissue is a house, is to see what can happen to people who inject steroids to gain muscle mass. They're using the injection to ask the connective tissue to "house" more muscle tissue. If you've ever seen some of these people who do this, you know how gigantic they can get. But sometimes, after years of use, the connective tissue gets confused, and instead of housing muscle tissue, it starts to house calcium. The end product is called an ossifican.

22

As you can see in this picture, the connective tissue has become confused from the steroids, and instead of housing muscle, it's housing calcium! The ossifican still looks like the striated muscle tissue, but it's "bone". And if you were to put this whole thing into vinegar for a month, like the chicken bone, the calcium would dissolve out and it would just be bendy connective tissue.

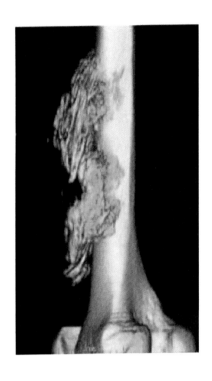

The last part of the house analogy deals with the immune system. Our connective tissue, which holds in all our guts and keeps our skin stuck to us, has a thin layer called the lamina propria. The lamina propria is where our immune system does its thing. In Traditional Chinese Medicine, we say that our defensive qi (wei qi) flows just under the skin, and that without good zheng qi (upright, chest, correct qi), wei qi won't be as good.

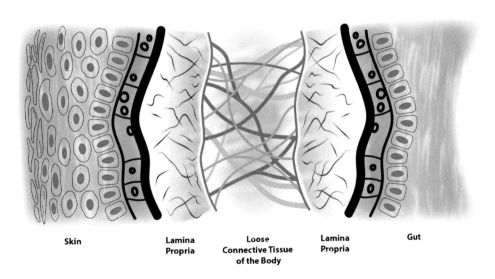

| Skin | Lamina Propria | Loose Connective Tissue of the Body | Lamina Propria | Gut |

While the lamina propria is greatly thickened in this illustration, it's part of the connective tissue, and if you're not squeezing that connective tissue through proper posture and walking, then you're allowing your immune system to be "lamina inapropria". Without all that amazing piezoelectric current strengthening our immune system, you start having inappropriate immune responses, and since there's a lamina propria connected to the gut, you start having immune reactions to foods that shouldn't have an immune reaction.

Nuts and gluten are perfect examples. The first generation of swaybacks had little immune issues, but my generation (the second swayback generation) had asthma here and there. My daughter's generation is besieged with immune problems – as well as other connective tissue problems like huge numbers of concussions, fastest growing rate of stroke, and rampant mental illness because the brain is 90% connective tissue.

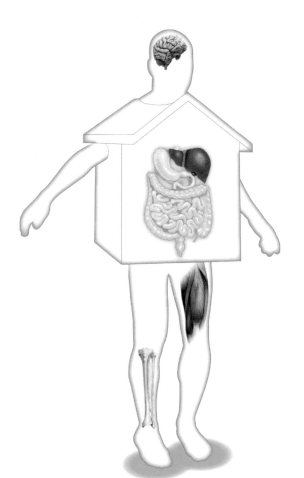

To bring all of these things together, I'd like to look at space, and what happens to humans that go into space. Aside from lengthening, they have no engagement of their connective tissue; they have no tensegrity. So, the first thing astronauts are faced with is Space Fever, which is an elevated temperature from the lamina propria not having any piezoelectric currents to help regulate it. Second, after a few weeks without piezoelectric current, their bones become brittle – much like swaybacks on earth with osteoporosis, but many, many times faster. Finally, if the astronauts aren't doing resistance work or some kind of exercise that mimics gravity (squeezing their connective tissue – they exercise two and a half hours a day, by the way), they end up with Space Brain, which is just a form dementia.

Make your house strong, and everything it houses will follow suit – don't be a swayback!

CHAPTER 9

Future Studies

Having seen so many people with weak cores in the modern world, and seeing how a lack of anatomical stability is rampant in the modern world, I'd love to see further studies done on the practice of forefoot walking in relation to strength, resilience, and even mindfulness.

The National Institute of Health published an amazing amount of research on loss of resiliency and lack of core strength with regard to erectile dysfunction, and lack of core strength with regard to incontinence.

I'd love to see someone do research on how changing to a primal walk may bring about changes with regard to infertility, endometriosis, enlarged prostate, and low testosterone from lack of blood flow and muscle development in the pelvic floor. I also think that people in the midst of joint-replacement surgery recovery would benefit by the loss of biostatic shock (the result of heel-striking as it is expressed in Lieberman et al. 2010). Since primal walking develops concentration and focus, I'd like to see it factored into research on ADD, ADHD, and behavioral problems in children and adults. Just as the IQ test results of some children's IQs are affected after the children are diagnosed with eye problems and they begin to wear glasses, IQ may also be affected by gait.

I'd also like to see research done on primal walking and teeth. It turns out that dentin and enamel are also piezoelectric, and since they are housed by the connective tissue as well, I would think that walking correctly would lead to straighter and stronger teeth. When you look at fossil records, our ancestors had straight teeth – and they walked right, too! Seeing how primal walking affects our telomere lengths would also be of interest – it turns out DNA is also piezoelectric.

We already know from NASA studies that piezoelectric current helps make bones grow, but I'd like to see how primal walking affects osteoporosis, dementia, and immune disorders.

Finally, I'd like to see how primal walking affects babies still in the womb (after they come out, of course). If a mother is walking correctly, she's generating huge amounts of piezoelectric currents, and those currents are going through her baby (not to mention that she's kneading/squeezing/hugging her child as she stands and walks correctly). Since those currents drive healthy tissue growth, the mother is strengthening her child even as the baby's developing inside her!

At times I feel like the guy in the 1940s telling others that smoking isn't good for them, but now we all know the long term bad effects smoking has on us. Imagine a culture that gives cigarettes to children as young as 2. When people in that culture reach their 50s, they start dying of lung cancer and emphysema. And everyone would just say that's part of getting old. But from our perspective, we'd say it's from smoking and that all those people could be so much more if they'd just stop smoking.

As long as we're open to examining what we hold as truth, we're in a position to grow and become stronger. What makes us the top mammals on the planet is our ability to change and adapt. As far as heel-striking goes, I would apply the old saying, "Just because we can doesn't mean we should."

CHAPTER 10

Summary

Now that you've read the book, here's a quick guide to help you in your path to maximized stability!

1. Put 99 percent or more of your weight on your forefoot with your hips over the balls of your feet and your knees loose.

2. Keep your head back so that your ears are in line with your shoulders.

3. Pull your chin in slightly (you should be looking straight ahead).

4. Don't worry about the shoulders—that is, don't pull them back.

5. Lift the chest/breastbone.

6. When you're walking, take shorter steps while landing on the forefoot.

Throughout the process, stay relaxed. While you may feel like you're tiptoeing for several months, it will eventually feel natural, and you'll come to love the strong core and tight stomach that this walk brings – not to mention the generation of all the piezoelectric current. It took me eight months before I felt like my walk was normal. The only way to accomplish it is to practice it, and the only way to practice it is to stay aware of how you're walking. The thinner the sole of your shoe, the better! Keeping on your toes and being on the ball aren't just expressions; they're a way of life.

About the Author

Author Greg Shim, LAc, MEd, is someone who doesn't know there ever existed a box outside of which to think. A husband and father, the licensed acupuncturist is also a woodworker, handyman, teacher, gourmet cook, and musician wannabe. Follow him on Instagram @primalwalk and on YouTube at Primal Walk.

For demonstrations and lectures about primal walking, contact Greg at greg@primalwalk.com.

Joe Walker can be reached at joe-walker.com

References

Cunningham C., N. Schilling, C. Anders, et al. 2010. "The Influence of Foot Posture on the Cost of Transport in Humans." Journal of Experimental Biology 213: 790–97.

Lieberman D. E., M. Venkadesan, W. A. Werbel, A. I. Daoud, S. D'Andrea, I. S. Davis, R. O. Mang'eni, and Y. Pitsiladis. 2010. "Foot Strike Patterns and Collision Forces in Habitually Barefoot versus Shod Runners." Nature 463: 531–35.

Official Statistics of Finland (OSF): Causes of death [e-publication].
ISSN=1799-5078. 2010, 2. Mortality from diseases in 1936 to 2010 . Helsinki: Statistics Finland [referred: 24.2.2018].
Access method: http://www.stat.fi/til/ksyyt/2010/ksyyt_2010_2011-12-16_kat_003_en.html

Kannus P, Parkkari J, Niemi S, Palvanen M. Epidemiology of Osteoporotic Ankle Fractures in Elderly Persons in Finland. Ann Intern Med. 1996;125:975–978. doi: 10.7326/0003-4819-125-12-199612150-00007

Pollack, S. R.; Korostoff, E.; Starkebaum,, W.; Lannicone,, W. (1979). "Micro-Electrical Studies of Stress-Generated Potentials in Bone". In Brighton, C. T.; Black, J.; Pollack, S. R. Electrical Properties of Bone and Cartilage. New York, NY: Grune & Stratton. ISBN 0-8089-1228-3.

Kissela BM1, Khoury JC, Alwell K, Moomaw CJ, Woo D, Adeoye O, Flaherty ML, Khatri P, Ferioli S, De Los Rios La Rosa F, Broderick JP, Kleindorfer DO. "Age at stroke: temporal trends in stroke incidence in a large, biracial population." Neurology. 2012 Oct 23;79(17):1781-7. doi: 10.1212/WNL.0b013e318270401d. Epub 2012 Oct 10.

American Academy of Neurology. "Physically fit women nearly 90 percent less likely to develop dementia." ScienceDaily. ScienceDaily, 15 March 2018. <www.sciencedaily.com/releases/2018/03/180315101805.htm>.

Niharika Arora Duggal, Ross D. Pollock, Norman R. Lazarus, Stephen Harridge, Janet M. Lord. First published: 8 March 2018. "Major features of immunesenescence, including reduced thymic output, are ameliorated by high levels of physical activity in adulthood". <https://doi.org/10.1111/acel.12750>

Made in the USA
San Bernardino, CA
07 August 2018